KRISTA BONDS

CHAIR YOGA

FOR SENIORS OVER 60

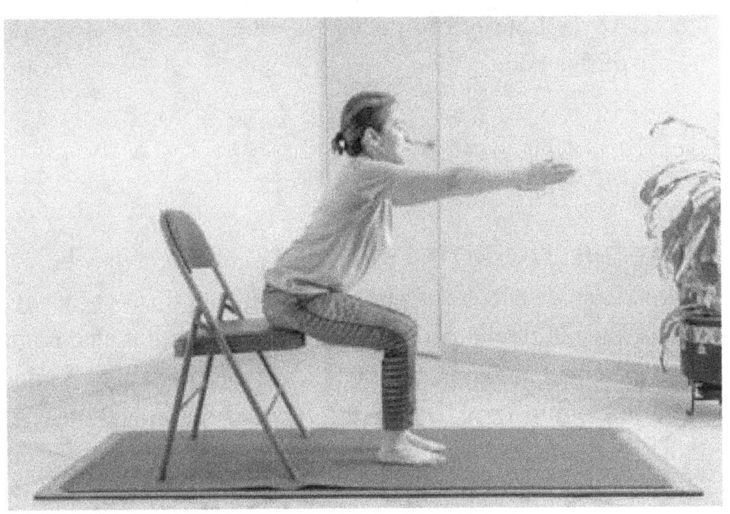

*Quick 10-Minute Chair Exercises for Seniors -
Regain Independence by Increasing Mobility &
Flexibility*

<u>DISCLAIMER</u>

The content provided in this book is for informational purposes only. The author is not responsible for any errors, omissions, or actions that may result from using the information contained in this book. All reasonable efforts have been taken to offer accurate, current, and comprehensive information. We recommend verifying all information before beginning any new exercise program, especially if you have health concerns and consulting with a qualified professional. The reader assumes all responsibility and risk associated with the use of this book.

Contents

Introduction

In the rhythmic dance of life, the pursuit of wellness is an everlasting melody. As we gracefully age, the symphony takes on new nuances, inviting us to explore pathways that blend movement, tranquility, and self-discovery. In this orchestration of well-being, Chair Yoga emerges as a transformative composition, designed for the seasoned souls seeking vitality and independence.

Welcome to **"Chair Yoga For Seniors Over 60: Quick 10-Minute Chair Exercises for Seniors - Regain Independence by Increasing Mobility & Flexibility."** I am thrilled to be your guide on this journey towards a more vibrant and resilient you. As the author, I too have traversed the winding roads of aging, recognizing the importance of embracing our bodies with compassion and empowering them with purpose.

In these pages, you'll discover not just a collection of exercises but a gateway to a renewed sense of self. The very essence of this book lies in the marriage of ancient yogic wisdom and the pragmatic needs of today's seniors. Through personal experiences, I've come to understand the profound impact that dedicated, yet accessible, chair yoga routines can have on our physical, mental, and emotional well-being.

Our voyage begins with a testament to the myriad benefits of chair yoga—more than just a series of poses, it's a holistic approach to aging gracefully. From enhanced mobility to the nurturing of independence, this practice beckons us to redefine what is possible at any age.

Together, we'll explore the fundamentals of chair yoga, creating a safe and enriching space within the comfort of your home. The carefully curated warm-up sequences and invigorating poses will not only bring flexibility to your limbs but also infuse vitality into your spirit. Beyond the physical, we delve into advanced practices that challenge and uplift, fostering strength and resilience.

This book is not a mere guide; it's a companion on your journey to rediscovering the joy of movement and the peace found in stillness. Embedded within its pages is a two-week workout plan—a roadmap to consistency and progress. Each day offers a ten-minute oasis of self-care, a commitment to your well-being that transcends the limitations of time.

As we embark on this odyssey together, remember that the chair beneath you is not just a seat; it is a vessel for transformation. Whether you are a seasoned yogi or a novice to the practice, these pages are crafted to meet you where you are and guide you toward where you want to be.

So, let the journey commence. Unroll your metaphorical mat, find solace in your chair, and let's embark on the empowering expedition of Chair Yoga—for it is not just about reclaiming movement; it's about reclaiming life.

Dive in, dear reader, and let the symphony of your own vitality begin.

The Benefits of Chair Yoga for Seniors - Enhancing Mobility and Independence

In the tapestry of aging, the quest for vitality takes center stage, and Chair Yoga emerges as a potent elixir, seamlessly weaving together the threads of physical well-being and independence. In this chapter, we unravel the rich tapestry of benefits that Chair Yoga unfurls for seniors, transcending the conventional notions of exercise and gracefully choreographing movements that enhance both mobility and independence.

Liberation Through Gentle Movement

Chair Yoga is a liberating dance for the body and spirit. As we gracefully age, our bodies may experience the tightening grip of stiffness and reduced mobility. Chair Yoga, with its gentle and adaptive postures, becomes the liberator—allowing the body to stretch, bend, and flow, irrespective of age or fitness level. Each movement is a step towards increased joint flexibility, ensuring that the body remains supple and responsive to the demands of daily life.

Empowering Independence in Every Pose

Independence is the cornerstone of a fulfilling life, and Chair Yoga becomes a beacon illuminating the path. Through a curated sequence of poses, this practice not only fosters physical independence but also cultivates a deep sense of self-reliance. Seniors find themselves empowered to perform daily activities with greater ease, from reaching for items on high shelves to navigating uneven terrain. Chair Yoga becomes a catalyst for breaking free from the perceived limitations of aging, fostering a renewed sense of capability.

Strengthening Core Stability

In the heart of Chair Yoga lies the nurturing of core stability. A strong core is the anchor that supports mobility and balance. Through intentional and controlled movements, seniors engage the core muscles, building strength that radiates outward, enhancing posture, and fortifying against the challenges of frailty. The chair becomes not just a prop but a steadfast partner in the journey to a more resilient and stable core.

Elevating Mood and Mental Clarity

Beyond the physical realm, Chair Yoga orchestrates a symphony of mental and emotional well-being. The rhythmic flow of movements, synchronized with conscious breathing, elicits a cascade of mood-elevating neurotransmitters. Seniors find respite from the challenges of aging, experiencing heightened mental clarity, reduced stress, and an overall sense of calm. Chair Yoga becomes a sanctuary—a refuge from the hustle of daily life, where the mind can find solace and rejuvenate.

In the fusion of gentle movements, empowering poses, and mindful breath, Chair Yoga becomes a transformative practice that transcends the boundaries of age. As we delve into the intricacies of its benefits, let us embark on a journey that not only enhances physical mobility but also liberates the spirit and nurtures the flame of independence, guiding seniors toward a life of grace, resilience, and fulfillment.

Chapter 1: Getting Started

1.1 Understanding Chair Yoga

Embarking on the Chair Yoga journey begins with a fundamental understanding of this transformative practice. Unlike traditional yoga, Chair Yoga provides an accessible and inclusive approach, making it an ideal companion for seniors seeking to reap the benefits of yoga without the need for complex floor exercises.

1.1.1 Adaptability for All Ages and Fitness Levels

Chair Yoga is a practice tailored to meet individuals where they are in their fitness journey. Its adaptability makes it suitable for seniors of all ages, abilities, and fitness levels. Whether you're a seasoned yogi or new to the practice, each pose is thoughtfully crafted to be approachable yet effective, ensuring that everyone can participate and experience the joy of movement.

1.1.2 Incorporating Mindfulness in Motion

At the core of Chair Yoga lies the marriage of movement and mindfulness. Each pose is an opportunity to cultivate a deep connection between body and mind. The emphasis on conscious breathwork intertwines with purposeful movements, creating a holistic experience that extends beyond the physical realm. As seniors engage in the practice, they find a tranquil space to center themselves, fostering a sense of inner peace and well-being.

1.2 Suitable Attire and Equipment

As we embark on this journey of self-discovery through Chair Yoga, selecting the right attire and equipment becomes a pivotal step toward creating a comfortable and enriching practice environment.

1.2.1 Comfort as a Priority

The essence of Chair Yoga lies in comfort. Opt for loose-fitting, breathable clothing that allows for unrestricted movement. Seniors are encouraged to choose attire that facilitates stretching and bending without constraint, ensuring a seamless and enjoyable practice.

1.2.2 The Supportive Role of a Sturdy Chair

Central to Chair Yoga is the utilization of a sturdy, stable chair. The chair serves as a reliable prop, offering support and balance throughout the practice. It becomes an extension of the practitioner, enabling a wide array of seated and standing poses. Choose a chair with a flat seat and a backrest for optimum comfort and stability.

1.2.3 Optional Props for Enhanced Experience

While a chair is a primary prop, additional accessories such as yoga blocks, cushions, and resistance bands can be incorporated to enhance the experience. These optional props provide added support and variety, allowing seniors to customize their practice to suit their individual needs and preferences.

In the realm of Chair Yoga, understanding the practice and selecting the right attire and equipment lay the foundation for a fulfilling and enriching experience. As we delve deeper into the subsequent chapters, remember that this practice is not just about physical movement; it is a holistic journey toward well-being, mindfulness, and self-discovery. So, let us take the first steps together, with comfort as our guide and the chair as our steadfast companion.

1.3 Safety First: Preparing Your Space

Ensuring a safe and secure practice environment is paramount in the Chair Yoga journey. This section guides you through the essential steps to create a space that fosters well-being and minimizes the risk of injury.

1.3.1 Clearing and Organizing Your Space

Begin by clearing the practice area of any potential hazards. Ensure that the space is clutter-free, with no obstacles that may impede movement or cause accidents. Organize the surroundings to create a dedicated space for your Chair Yoga practice, allowing you to move freely and with confidence.

1.3.2 Adequate Lighting for Clarity

Proper lighting is kcy to a safe practice. Ensure that the practice space is well-lit, minimizing shadows and creating a clear visual environment. Adequate lighting not only reduces the risk of tripping or missteps but also enhances your focus on the poses and movements, promoting a mindful and safe practice.

1.3.3 Secure Flooring for Stability

The surface beneath your chair should be stable and slip-resistant. Place your chair on a non-slip mat or a carpet to prevent any accidental sliding. This provides a secure foundation, especially during standing poses, ensuring stability and reducing the risk of slips or falls.

1.4 Tips for a Secure Practice

Navigating the nuances of Chair Yoga with safety in mind is a foundational step toward a fulfilling practice. The following tips offer guidance on how to approach your practice securely and confidently.

1.4.1 Listen to Your Body

Chair Yoga is a practice of self-awareness. Listen attentively to your body's signals and respect its limitations. If a pose feels uncomfortable or causes pain, modify or skip it. Honoring your body's cues fosters a safe and sustainable practice.

1.4.2 Utilize the Chair for Support

The chair is not just a prop; it's a reliable source of support. Use the chair's backrest and arms for balance and stability, especially during standing poses. This ensures a secure foundation and empowers you to explore a broader range of movements.

1.4.3 Gradual Progression Over Perfection

Embrace the journey of gradual progression. Chair Yoga is about building strength, flexibility, and balance over time. Avoid pushing yourself too hard and celebrate the small victories. Consistent and mindful practice yields more sustainable results than attempting overly challenging poses prematurely.

1.4.4 Warm-up Adequately

Prepare your body for the practice ahead by incorporating a gentle warm-up routine. Focus on neck and shoulder stretches, wrist and ankle circles, and deep breaths. Warming up primes your muscles and joints, reducing the risk of strain or injury during the main practice.

As we embark on this transformative journey, remember that safety is the cornerstone of a fulfilling Chair Yoga practice. By preparing your space thoughtfully and adhering to secure practices, you lay the groundwork for an enriching experience that fosters well-being, self-discovery, and the joy of movement. Let safety guide your practice, and may each pose unfold with confidence and ease.

Chapter 2: Quick Chair Warm-ups

2.1 Neck and Shoulder Exercises: Loosening Tension

In the art of Chair Yoga, the gateway to a rejuvenated practice lies in the mindful release of tension from the neck and shoulders. These gentle exercises serve as the prelude to a symphony of movement, allowing you to ease into your practice with grace and intention.

2.1.1 Neck Rolls: A Fluid Unwinding

Begin by sitting comfortably in your chair with your spine straight and shoulders relaxed. Inhale deeply, and as you exhale, lower your chin to your chest. Slowly rotate your head to the right, bringing your right ear toward your right shoulder. Inhale and return to the center, then exhale as you rotate to the left. Continue this fluid motion for 1-2 minutes, allowing your neck to unwind and release any accumulated tension.

2.1.2 Shoulder Shrug and Roll: Elevate, Relax, and Release

Sit with your feet flat on the ground, shoulders relaxed. Inhale deeply as you lift both shoulders toward your ears, holding for a moment. Exhale and roll your shoulders back and down in a circular motion. Repeat this sequence for 1-2 minutes, emphasizing the elevation, relaxation, and circular movement. This exercise promotes blood flow, alleviating tension in the shoulders.

2.1.3 Seated Cat-Cow Stretch: Mobilizing the Neck and Spine

Sit comfortably, ensuring your feet are flat on the ground. Inhale, arching your back and lifting your chest. Simultaneously, tilt your head back slightly, allowing a gentle stretch in the front of your neck. Exhale, rounding your spine and bringing your chin towards your chest. Repeat this cat-cow motion for 1-2 minutes, synchronizing breath with movement to enhance flexibility in the neck and spine.

2.1.4 Ear to Shoulder Stretch: Targeted Release

Sit tall, inhale, and as you exhale, lower your right ear toward your right shoulder, feeling a gentle stretch along the left side of your neck. Inhale back to center, and exhale as you switch to the left side. Repeat this stretch for 1-2 minutes, allowing the breath to guide the movement and deepen the stretch in each repetition.

2.1.5 Seated Neck Stretch: Embracing Serenity

Sit comfortably and extend your right arm down to the side of your chair. Inhale and lift your left arm, bringing it over your head, gently clasping your right ear. Exhale and tilt your head to the right, feeling a stretch along the left side of your neck. Hold for a few breaths, then switch sides. This seated neck stretch invites serenity and elongates the neck muscles.

Incorporating these neck and shoulder exercises into your Chair Yoga warm-up routine provides a gateway to enhanced mobility and a mindful beginning to your practice. Feel the tension melt away as you engage in these soothing movements, setting the stage for a harmonious exploration of the transformative power of Chair Yoga.

2.2 Wrist and Ankle Circles: Enhancing Joint Flexibility

In the intricate tapestry of Chair Yoga, the canvas of joint flexibility is painted with the rhythmic strokes of wrist and ankle circles. These simple yet powerful exercises serve as a cornerstone in priming the body for the flowing movements that follow, inviting you to embrace the symphony of mobility with grace and fluidity.

2.2.1 Wrist Circles: A Dance of Articulation

Begin by sitting comfortably, resting your hands on your thighs. Inhale deeply, and as you exhale, extend your right arm forward, forming a gentle fist. Rotate your wrist in a circular motion, gradually increasing the size of the circles. After a few rotations, switch to the left wrist. Continue this dance of articulation for 1-2 minutes, allowing the wrists to release tension and cultivate a sense of fluidity.

2.2.2 Ankle Circles: Grounded Elegance

Sit with your feet flat on the ground. Inhale as you lift your right foot slightly, circling your ankle clockwise. Exhale and circle the ankle counterclockwise. After a few rotations, switch to the left ankle. Repeat this grounded elegance for 1-2 minutes, fostering flexibility and awareness in the ankles. This exercise encourages a connection with the earth, grounding and stabilizing the lower body.

2.2.3 Combined Flow: Syncing Wrist and Ankle Circles

In a seamless fusion of movement, combine wrist circles with ankle circles for a synchronized flow. Inhale as you extend your right arm forward, initiating wrist circles. Simultaneously, lift your right foot, engaging in ankle circles. Exhale and transition to the left side. This integrated movement not only enhances joint flexibility but also cultivates coordination and balance. Flow through this combination for 2-3 minutes, immersing yourself in the fluidity of the interconnected circles.

2.2.4 Mindful Breath Integration

As you engage in wrist and ankle circles, weave the thread of conscious breath into the fabric of your movements. Inhale deeply during the upward motion, expanding the chest, and exhale fully as you complete the circle. This mindful breath integration not only enhances oxygenation but also establishes a serene rhythm, promoting a heightened sense of presence and focus.

2.2.5 Gentle Progression for Lasting Flexibility

In the realm of Chair Yoga, the emphasis is not on achieving perfection but on the gentle progression towards lasting flexibility. These wrist and ankle circles are not just exercises; they are invitations to explore the full range of motion within your body, fostering a sense of liberation and ease.

As we embark on the rhythmic journey of joint flexibility, let the circles become a dance—a celebration of the body's capacity for fluid movement. May the wrists and ankles lead the way, guiding you into a realm of enhanced mobility and a harmonious prelude to the unfolding practice of Chair Yoga.

Chapter 3: Seated Yoga Poses

3.1 Mountain Pose in a Chair: Focusing on Alignment

In the sanctuary of Chair Yoga, the iconic Mountain Pose finds its expression, grounded and majestic even within the confines of a chair. This seated adaptation invites practitioners to embark on a journey of alignment, strength, and mindful presence, bringing the essence of the mountain into the rhythm of their being.

3.1.1 Foundation of Stability

Begin by sitting with your feet planted firmly on the ground, hip-width apart. Imagine your feet as the base of the mountain, rooted and stable. Distribute your weight evenly across both feet, grounding yourself in the present moment. The chair becomes the bedrock, supporting your ascent into the mountain pose.

3.1.2 Spinal Elevation

Inhale deeply, elongating your spine as if a thread were gently pulling you upward from the crown of your head. Visualize the mountain's summit and allow your spine to reach towards it. The chair provides a supportive foundation for the spine's elevation, fostering a sense of openness and alignment.

3.1.3 Engaging Core Strength

As you ascend into the mountain, engage your core muscles gently. This subtle engagement creates a sense of stability, mirroring the strength of the mountain's core. The chair serves as a guide, allowing you to explore the activation of your abdominal muscles without strain.

3.1.4 Arm Alignment and Intentional Breath

Extend your arms alongside your body, palms facing inward. Align your arms with the intention of reaching towards the sky, mirroring the mountain's peaks. With each inhalation, feel the expansion in your chest and the elevation of your arms. As you exhale, release any tension, allowing the breath to guide the gentle ascent and descent.

3.1.5 Mindful Presence

Mountain Pose in a chair is not merely a physical alignment but a practice of mindful presence. Close your eyes if comfortable, or maintain a soft gaze forward. Feel the stillness and strength of the mountain within you. As thoughts arise, let them flow like the breeze around the mountain, acknowledging their presence without attachment.

3.1.6 Modifications for Comfort

Every mountain is unique, and so is every practitioner. Feel free to modify the pose to suit your comfort. If sitting for an extended period is challenging, consider placing a cushion or folded blanket under you for added support. The essence of the pose lies in the mindful alignment and connection to your inner strength.

3.1.7 Mountain Pose Visualization

As you hold the Mountain Pose in a chair, visualize yourself as the mountain—steadfast, unyielding, and deeply rooted. Connect with the symbolism of the mountain, embodying resilience and unwavering presence. In this seated rendition, the chair becomes not just a prop but a throne, inviting you to reign over your inner landscape with grace and poise.

Mountain Pose in a chair is an invitation to align with the innate strength within. As you embody the essence of the mountain, may you find stability in the present moment, strength in your core, and a heightened sense of mindful presence. In the symphony of Chair Yoga, let the Mountain Pose be a resounding note, echoing the harmonious balance of body, mind, and spirit.

3.2 Chair Sun Salutations: Energizing the Body

In the choreography of Chair Yoga, the rhythmic dance of Sun Salutations unfolds, bringing a burst of vitality and energy to the seated practitioner. Chair Sun Salutations become a fluid sequence, a dynamic celebration that harmonizes breath, movement, and intention—invigorating the body with the warmth of the sun's embrace.

3.2.1 Seated Mountain Pose: The Commencement

Begin in Seated Mountain Pose, your foundation rooted in the chair, spine elongated, and arms gracefully resting alongside your body. Inhale deeply, reach your arms overhead and exhale with intention. This opening salutation sets the stage for the energetic flow to follow.

3.2.2 Forward Fold with Graceful Arms: Embracing Surrender

On the next inhalation, hinge at your hips, leading with your heart, and fold forward. Allow your arms to sweep forward and down, mirroring the descent of the sun. Let your head hang gently, releasing any tension in your neck and shoulders. This forward fold embraces surrender, preparing for the renewed ascent.

3.2.3 Seated Extended Mountain Pose: Rising with Renewed Energy

Inhale, and with grace, lift your torso back up to the Seated Extended Mountain Pose. Feel the energizing stretch along your spine, embracing the renewed energy rising within you. Your arms extend overhead, reaching for the sky as if capturing the essence of the sun's warmth.

3.2.4 Seated Forward Bend: Grounding with Intention

Exhale and transition into a Seated Forward Bend, hands reaching toward your feet. Feel the grounding sensation as you bow forward, connecting with the Earth beneath you. This moment of groundedness prepares you for the next phase of the salutation.

3.2.5 Seated Mountain Pose with a Twist: Radiating Energy

Inhale and return to Seated Mountain Pose, this time introducing a gentle twist. Place your right hand on your left knee and your left hand on the back of the chair, twisting your torso to the left. Feel the gentle wringing out of tension as you radiate energy outward.

3.2.6 Repeat on the Other Side: Balanced Harmony

Exhale and return to the center, then repeat the seated twist on the other side. This balanced harmony embodies the cyclical nature of the Sun Salutations, inviting symmetry and equilibrium into your practice.

3.2.7 Concluding in Seated Mountain Pose: A Moment of Stillness

Finish the sequence by returning to Seated Mountain Pose, basking in the warmth and energy cultivated throughout the salutation. Take a few breaths, acknowledge the vitality coursing through your body, and revel in the sense of renewal and invigoration.

Chair Sun Salutations are a symphony of movement, breath, and energy—a celebration of the sun's life-giving power within the framework of a seated practice. As you flow through this dynamic sequence, may you feel the revitalizing embrace of the sun, awakening a vibrant energy that permeates every fiber of your being. In the luminosity of Chair Sun Salutations, discover a sanctuary of vitality and a harmonious dance with the radiant source of life.

3.3 Seated Forward Bend Variations: Stretching the Back and Hamstrings

Within the tranquil landscape of Chair Yoga, the Seated Forward Bend beckons practitioners into a gentle symphony of flexibility and release. These variations of the classic pose offer a nuanced exploration of stretching the back and hamstrings, inviting a graceful journey into the depths of each bend.

3.3.1 Basic Seated Forward Bend: Nurturing the Foundation

Commence in a seated position at the edge of your chair, feet planted firmly on the ground. Inhale deeply, lengthening your spine, and exhale as you hinge at your hips, gently folding forward. Let your hands reach towards your feet or rest on your shins, allowing the stretch to cascade along your back and hamstrings. Hold this foundational pose for 30 seconds to a minute, breathing deeply into the stretch.

3.3.2 Supported Seated Forward Bend: Embracing Stability

For added support, place a yoga block or cushion on your lap. Inhale, elongate your spine and exhale into the forward fold. Rest your hands on the block or cushion, allowing your upper body to surrender with support. This variation provides stability and is particularly beneficial for those seeking a gentler approach to the stretch.

3.3.3 One-Legged Seated Forward Bend: Targeted Stretch

Inhale and extend your right leg forward while keeping your left foot firmly planted. Exhale as you hinge forward, directing your stretch toward the extended leg. This one-legged variation targets specific areas, intensifying the stretch along the back and hamstrings of the extended leg. Hold for 30 seconds, then switch to the other leg.

3.3.4 Seated Forward Bend with Twist: Unwinding Tension

Inhale and return to the basic seated forward bend. Exhale as you introduce a gentle twist to the right, bringing your left hand to the outside of your right knee. Feel the twist through your spine, unlocking tension in the back. Inhale back to center and exhale into a twist on the left side. This variation adds a therapeutic element, aiding in the release of tension along the entire back.

3.3.5 Seated Forward Bend with Shoulder Opener: Expanding the Stretch

Begin in the basic seated forward bend. As you fold forward, interlace your fingers behind your back and extend your arms overhead. This variation not only deepens the stretch in your back and hamstrings but also opens the shoulders, fostering a sense of expansiveness. Hold for 30 seconds, allowing the stretch to radiate through your upper body.

3.3.6 Dynamic Seated Forward Bend Flow: Embracing Fluidity

Combine the variations into a dynamic flow. Inhale to the basic seated forward bend, exhale into a one-legged stretch, inhale back to center, and exhale into a twist. Allow the movements to flow seamlessly, creating a dance of flexibility and release. This dynamic flow not only stretches the back and hamstrings but also encourages a sense of fluidity in your practice.

In the poetic tapestry of Chair Yoga, the Seated Forward Bend Variations are verses of flexibility and release. Each variation invites practitioners to explore the subtle nuances of the stretch, fostering a deep connection with the body's unfolding grace. As you gracefully move through these variations, may you discover the symphony of suppleness, a melody that resonates through the back and hamstrings, enriching your practice with each bend and release.

3.4 Seated Twist Sequence: Promoting Spinal Health

In the sanctuary of Chair Yoga, the Seated Twist Sequence emerges as a gentle yet powerful melody, weaving through the spine and promoting a symphony of spinal health. These variations of seated twists invite practitioners to harmonize breath, movement, and intention, fostering a nurturing dance that revitalizes the spine.

3.4.1 Seated Twist to the Right: Initiating the Sequence

Begin seated at the edge of your chair, spine tall and shoulders relaxed. Inhale deeply, and as you exhale, initiate the twist to the right. Place your left hand on your right knee and your right hand on the backrest of the chair. Feel the gentle rotation through your spine, elongating and promoting flexibility. Hold for 30 seconds, focusing on the rhythm of your breath.

3.4.2 Seated Twist to the Left: Balancing the Sequence

Inhale back to the center, allowing your spine to reset. Exhale into the twist on the left side, placing your right hand on your left knee and your left hand on the backrest. Embrace the sensation of the twist, feeling the revitalization coursing through your spine. Hold for 30 seconds, breathing into the depth of the stretch.

3.4.3 Seated Twist with Shoulder Opener: Expanding the Movement

As you twist to the right, extend your left arm across your body, reaching for the backrest of the chair. This addition opens the shoulders and enhances the stretch along the spine. Inhale back to center, and exhale into the twist on the left side, extending your right arm. This expansion of movement not only promotes spinal health but also invites a delightful stretch through the shoulders.

3.4.4 Seated Twist Flow: Embracing Fluidity

Combine the twists into a seamless flow. Inhale to the center, exhale into the twist on the right, inhale back to the center, and exhale into the twist on the left. Allow the movements to unfold with grace and fluidity, creating a continuous dance that revitalizes the spine and fosters a sense of balance. This dynamic flow can be repeated for 2-3 minutes, immersing yourself in the rhythmic sequence.

3.4.5 Chair Eagle Pose: Enhancing the Twist

Bring a playful variation to the Seated Twist Sequence with Chair Eagle Pose. Cross your right thigh over the left, then wrap your left foot around your right calf. As you twist to the right, bring your left elbow over your right knee. This seated variation of Eagle Pose deepens the twist, promoting spinal flexibility and integrity. Inhale back to center and repeat on the left side.

3.4.6 Seated Twist with Forward Fold: Integrating Depth

Begin in the basic seated position. Inhale and elongate your spine, then exhale into a twist to the right. From this twist, extend your torso forward, reaching your hands toward the right foot. This integrated movement combines the benefits of a twist with a forward fold, promoting both spinal health and hamstring flexibility. Inhale back to center and repeat on the left side.

The Seated Twist Sequence in Chair Yoga is an exploration of the spine's profound capacity for movement and rejuvenation. Each twist is a note in the composition of spinal health, inviting practitioners to embrace the fluidity and grace inherent in the dance of the spine. As you engage in this sequence, you may feel the revitalizing rhythm of the twists, fostering a resilient and supple spine that harmonizes with the melody of your breath and movement.

Chapter 4: Advanced Chair Yoga

4.1 Seated Warrior Poses: Building Strength and Stability

In the refined realm of Chair Yoga, the Seated Warrior Poses stand as formidable sentinels—guardians of strength, stability, and inner fortitude. These advanced variations echo the warrior spirit, inviting practitioners to embrace a deeper exploration of their physical and mental capabilities within the sanctuary of their chairs.

4.1.1 Seated Warrior I: Grounding and Expanding

Commence by sitting tall on the edge of your chair, feet firmly planted on the ground. Inhale deeply, lifting your arms overhead. As you exhale, bring your right foot back, grounding the sole into the floor. Engage your core and feel the expansion through your chest and arms, embodying the strength of a warrior. Hold for 30 seconds to a minute, then switch to the left side.

4.1.2 Seated Warrior II: Dynamic Alignment

From Seated Warrior I, open your hips and shoulders to the side, extending your arms parallel to the ground. The right knee remains bent, aligning over the ankle, while the left foot continues to ground firmly. This dynamic alignment not only builds strength in the lower body but also encourages a sense of openness and readiness. Hold for 30 seconds to a minute, then transition to the left side.

4.1.3 Seated Warrior III: Balancing Elegance

Seated Warrior III introduces an element of balance and elegance to the sequence. Begin in Seated Warrior I, then hinge forward at the hips, lifting your right leg parallel to the ground while extending your arms forward. The body forms a T shape, cultivating strength in the core and stability in the supporting leg. Hold for 30 seconds to a minute before switching to the left side.

4.1.4 Seated Reverse Warrior: Expanding the Horizon

Incorporate a gentle backbend into the warrior sequence with Seated Reverse Warrior. From Seated Warrior II, maintain the bend in the right knee and reach your left arm overhead, creating a graceful arc. Feel the expansion through the left side of your body, fostering flexibility and strength. Hold for 30 seconds to a minute, then transition to the left side.

4.1.5 Seated Warrior Flow: A Dynamic Symphony

Combine the Seated Warrior Poses into a fluid sequence. Inhale to Seated Warrior I, exhale to Seated Warrior II, inhale to Seated Warrior III, and exhale to Seated Reverse Warrior. Allow the movements to flow seamlessly, creating a dynamic symphony of strength, stability, and grace. This flow can be repeated for 2-3 minutes, embodying the spirit of a warrior in motion.

4.1.6 Seated Eagle Pose: Integrating Strength and Balance

Bring a fusion of strength and balance to the Seated Warrior sequence with Seated Eagle Pose. From Seated Warrior II, cross your right thigh over the left, then wrap your left foot around your right calf. Bring your palms together in front of your heart, emulating the embrace of an eagle. This seated variation builds strength in the legs and enhances balance. Hold for 30 seconds to a minute before switching sides.

4.1.7 Warrior Visualization Meditation: Embracing Inner Strength

Conclude the Seated Warrior sequence with a brief meditation. Close your eyes and envision yourself as a warrior—strong, resilient, and grounded. With each breath, inhale the energy of a warrior, and as you exhale, release any tension or self-doubt. This visualization meditation enhances the mental and emotional aspects of the warrior spirit.

Seated Warrior Poses in advanced Chair Yoga is an embodiment of strength, stability, and inner fortitude. As you engage in these variations, may you feel the warrior within, standing tall and unyielding in the face of life's challenges. Let the chair be your throne, and each pose a testament to the power that resides within you—a warrior, poised, and graceful in the dance of strength and stability.

4.2 Leg Lifts and Extensions: Enhancing Lower Body Strength

In the dynamic landscape of Chair Yoga, Leg Lifts and Extensions emerge as sculptors of lower body strength—a testament to the transformative power within the embrace of your chair. These exercises not only fortify the muscles but also cultivate balance, flexibility, and a profound connection with the foundation that supports you.

4.2.1 Seated Leg Lifts: Elevating Strength

Sit tall on the edge of your chair, feet flat on the ground. Inhale deeply, engage your core and lift your right leg straight in front of you. Hold for a moment, then exhale and lower it back down. Repeat on the left side. The controlled movement of Seated Leg Lifts targets the quadriceps and engages the core, enhancing lower body strength. Perform 10-15 repetitions on each leg.

4.2.2 Seated Leg Extensions: Unleashing Potential

Building on the foundation of Seated Leg Lifts, progress to Seated Leg Extensions for a more extended range of motion. Inhale as you lift your right leg, and then exhale as you extend it forward, reaching for the toes. Inhale back to the starting position, and exhale to lower the leg. Repeat on the left side. This dynamic extension not only strengthens the legs but also encourages flexibility. Aim for 10-15 repetitions on each leg.

4.2.3 Seated Cross-Leg Lifts: Engaging Inner Thighs

Sit with your spine straight and your knees bent. Inhale deeply, lift your right foot and cross it over your left knee. Exhale as you extend the right leg forward, engaging the inner thighs. Inhale back to the crossed position, and exhale to lower the leg. Repeat on the left side. Seated Cross-Leg Lifts target the inner thighs, promoting balanced lower body strength. Perform 10-15 repetitions on each leg.

4.2.4 Seated Side Leg Lifts: Lateral Power

Sit with your spine tall and both feet flat on the ground. Inhale deeply, lift your right leg and exhale as you extend it to the side. Inhale back to the center, and exhale to lower the leg. Repeat on the left side. Seated Side Leg Lifts engage the outer thighs, enhancing lateral strength. Aim for 10-15 repetitions on each leg.

4.2.5 Seated Figure-Four Leg Lifts: Balancing Act

Sit with your feet flat on the ground, knees bent. Inhale as you lift your right leg, and exhale as you cross it over your left knee, forming a figure-four shape. Inhale to lift the crossed leg, engaging the glutes and outer thighs. Exhale to lower the leg. Repeat on the left side. Seated Figure-Four Leg Lifts not only strengthen the lower body but also challenge balance. Perform 10-15 repetitions on each leg.

4.2.6 Seated Bicycle Legs: Dynamic Motion

Sit comfortably with your hands resting on the sides of the chair. Inhale as you lift your right leg and bring the knee toward your chest, mimicking a cycling motion. Exhale as you extend the right leg straight. Inhale to bring it back to the chest, and exhale to lower the leg. Repeat on the left side. Seated Bicycle Legs combine strength and dynamic movement, targeting the entire lower body. Aim for 10-15 repetitions on each leg.

4.2.7 Seated Leg Lifts and Extensions Flow: Fluid Strength

Combine the various leg lifts and extensions into a flowing sequence. Inhale for the lift, exhale for the extension and find a rhythm that feels natural. The fluidity of this flow not only enhances lower body strength but also invites a meditative quality into the movements. Perform the flow for 2-3 minutes, embracing the union of strength, breath, and motion.

Leg Lifts and Extensions in advanced Chair Yoga are a gateway to unlocking the potential of your lower body strength. As you engage in these exercises, may you feel the vitality coursing through your legs, grounding you in the strength that emanates from the foundation of your chair. Let each lift and extension be a testament to the resilience and power that resides within—the embodiment of a harmonious dance with strength and grace.

4.3 Dynamic Chair Yoga Flow: Integrating Fluid Movements

In the symphony of advanced Chair Yoga, the Dynamic Chair Yoga Flow takes center stage—a captivating dance that seamlessly integrates fluid movements, breath, and mindfulness. This dynamic sequence transcends the confines of static poses, inviting practitioners into a rhythmic exploration that harmonizes strength, flexibility, and inner serenity.

4.3.1 Seated Cat-Cow Flow: Initiating Fluidity

Begin in a comfortable seated position with your hands on your thighs. Inhale, arching your back, and lifting your chest (Seated Cow Pose). Exhale, rounding your spine and bringing your chin to your chest (Seated Cat Pose). Continue this flowing movement, synchronizing breath with motion. The

Seated Cat-Cow Flow serves as the foundation, initiating the fluidity of the sequence. Repeat for 1-2 minutes.

4.3.2 Seated Sun Salutations: Embracing Vitality

From Seated Cat-Cow, flow into Seated Sun Salutations. Inhale, reaching your arms overhead, and exhale, bringing your hands to the heart center. Inhale to lift your arms again, and exhale to release them back down. This dynamic variation of Sun Salutations energizes the body, fostering a sense of vitality and warmth. Repeat for 2-3 minutes, allowing the movements to unfold with grace.

4.3.3 Seated Warrior Flow: Channeling Inner Strength

Transition into the Seated Warrior Flow. Inhale to Seated Warrior I, exhale to Seated Warrior II, inhale to Seated Warrior III, and exhale to Seated Reverse Warrior. Allow the movements to flow seamlessly, embodying the strength and grace of a warrior in motion. This dynamic sequence not only builds physical strength but also channels inner resilience. Repeat for 2-3 minutes.

4.3.4 Seated Twist and Reach: Spiraling Grace

From the warrior flow, transition into Seated Twist and Reach. Inhale as you twist to the right, reaching your left hand to the outside of the right knee. Exhale back to center, and inhale to twist to the left, reaching your right hand to the outside of the left knee. This spiraling motion enhances spinal flexibility and grace. Repeat for 1-2 minutes.

4.3.5 Seated Forward Bend Flow: Folding with Intention

Move into a Seated Forward Bend Flow by inhaling to lift your arms overhead and exhaling into a forward fold. Inhale to lift back up, and exhale to lower your hands. This flowing sequence not only stretches the spine and hamstrings but also encourages a meditative connection with breath and movement. Repeat for 2-3 minutes, finding a rhythm of folding and unfolding.

4.3.6 Dynamic Leg Lifts and Extensions: Power and Fluidity

Incorporate Dynamic Leg Lifts and Extensions into the flow. Inhale for the lift, exhale for the extension, and seamlessly transition between legs. This addition infuses the flow with power and fluidity, enhancing lower body strength and balance. Continue for 2-3 minutes, feeling the rhythmic engagement of your legs.

4.3.7 Seated Tree Pose Flow: Finding Balance

Conclude the Dynamic Chair Yoga Flow with a Seated Tree Pose Flow. Inhale to lift your right foot, placing it on the inner left thigh. Exhale to lower it back down. Inhale to lift the left foot, placing it on the inner right thigh. Exhale to lower. This balancing flow brings a sense of grounded serenity to the sequence. Repeat for 1-2 minutes.

The Dynamic Chair Yoga Flow is an invitation to immerse yourself in the fluidity of movement—a dance that transcends the boundaries of traditional yoga poses. As you gracefully navigate through each transition, may you find a profound connection between breath, body, and the present moment. In this dynamic flow, discover the beauty of integrating fluid movements, fostering a harmonious union of strength, flexibility, and inner peace within the embrace of your chair.

Chapter 5: Balance and Relaxation

5.1 Chair-Assisted Standing Poses: Improving Balance

In the tranquil realm of Chair Yoga's Balance and Relaxation chapter, Chair-Assisted Standing Poses emerge as gentle guides toward enhanced stability and poise. Rooted in the support of a chair, these poses provide a secure foundation for practitioners to explore and elevate their sense of balance with grace and confidence.

5.1.1 Chair Mountain Pose: Anchoring Stability

Begin by standing tall behind the chair, feet hip-width apart. Inhale deeply, reaching your arms overhead, palms facing each other. Engage your core and ground your feet firmly on the floor. The chair serves as a steady companion, offering support as you embody the essence of the mountain. Hold for 30 seconds to a minute, breathing into the stability of Chair Mountain Pose.

5.1.2 Chair Tree Pose: Rooted Elegance

Stand beside the chair, holding onto the backrest with your right hand. Shift your weight to your left leg and place the sole of your right foot against the inner left thigh or calf. Find your balance and bring your palms together at the heart center. The chair provides gentle support as you embrace the elegance of Chair Tree Pose. Hold for 30 seconds to a minute on each leg.

5.1.3 Chair Warrior Pose: Graceful Strength

Face the chair, placing your hands on the backrest for support. Step your right foot back, keeping the heel lifted and toes pointing forward. Bend your left knee, aligning it over the ankle. Engage your core and lift your arms overhead, creating a gentle backbend. Chair Warrior Pose embodies strength and grace, supported by the chair. Hold for 30 seconds to a minute, then switch legs.

5.1.4 Chair Dancer Pose: Fluid Alignment

Stand behind the chair, holding onto the backrest with both hands. Shift your weight to your left leg and bend your right knee, bringing the heel toward the buttocks. Reach your right hand back and hold onto the inside of your right foot. Allow your left arm to extend forward, maintaining a fluid line of alignment. Chair Dancer Pose harmonizes balance and flexibility. Hold for 30 seconds to a minute on each side.

5.1.5 Chair Side Plank: Core Stability

Place your hands on the backrest of the chair, arms extended. Step your feet back, aligning them with your hips. Engage your core and lift your body, creating a straight line from head to heels. The Chair Side Plank offers a gentle introduction to the traditional pose, emphasizing core stability with the aid of the chair. Hold for 30 seconds to a minute on each side.

5.1.6 Chair Eagle Pose: Balanced Integration

Stand beside the chair, holding onto the backrest with your right hand. Cross your left thigh over the right, then hook the left foot behind the right calf. Bring your palms together in front of your heart. Chair Eagle Pose seamlessly integrates balance and concentration, supported by the chair. Hold for 30 seconds to a minute on each side.

5.1.7 Chair-Assisted Standing Forward Fold: Grounding Release

Stand with your feet hip-width apart, holding onto the backrest of the chair. Inhale to lengthen your spine, and exhale as you hinge at the hips, folding forward. Allow your head to hang freely. The chair provides a stable base, allowing you to experience the grounding release of the Chair-Assisted Standing Forward Fold. Hold for 30 seconds to a minute.

Chair-Assisted Standing Poses are gateways to improved balance, offering a supportive transition from seated to standing postures. As you gracefully integrate these poses into your practice, may the chair become a steadfast companion on your journey toward enhanced stability, balance, and a profound sense of well-being. Each pose is an opportunity to explore the dance of balance, enveloped in the soothing embrace of your chair.

5.2 Cool Down and Guided Relaxation: Meditation Techniques for Seniors

As we transition into the soothing finale of our Chair Yoga journey, the Cool Down and Guided Relaxation chapter becomes a sanctuary for rejuvenation and serenity. Tailored specifically for seniors, these meditation techniques offer a gentle repose, guiding practitioners into a state of deep relaxation, mindful breath, and inner tranquility.

5.2.1 Seated Breath Awareness: Calming the Mind

Find a comfortable seated position, hands resting on your thighs. Close your eyes and turn your attention to your breath. Inhale deeply, feeling the expansion of your chest and abdomen. Exhale slowly, releasing tension. With each breath, invite a sense of calm to envelop you. Continue this seated breath awareness for 3-5 minutes, allowing the soothing rhythm to calm the mind.

5.2.2 Body Scan Meditation: Releasing Tension

Remain seated with your eyes closed. Direct your focus to different parts of your body, starting from your toes and moving upward. As you scan each area, inhale to bring awareness, and exhale to release any tension or tightness. This Body Scan Meditation promotes a sense of relaxation and heightened body awareness. Take 5-7 minutes to complete the scan, savoring the release with each breath.

5.2.3 Guided Visualization: Nature's Retreat

Close your eyes and envision a serene natural setting—a peaceful garden, a tranquil beach, or a calming forest. Engage your senses by imagining the sights, sounds, and scents of this retreat. As you breathe deeply, immerse yourself in the tranquility of your chosen visualization. Allow the serene imagery to wash away any remaining stress or worry. Spend 5-7 minutes in this guided visualization, absorbing the rejuvenating energy of nature.

5.2.4 Loving-Kindness Meditation: Cultivating Compassion

Return to a comfortable seated position and bring to mind someone you care about deeply—a friend, family member, or even yourself. Inhale, feeling love and warmth fill your heart. Exhale, extending this love outward. Repeat phrases like "May you be happy, may you be healthy, may you be at ease." Extend these wishes to others and, ultimately, to all beings. Loving-Kindness Meditation fosters a sense of compassion and connection. Practice for 5-7 minutes, embracing the expansive nature of loving-kindness.

5.2.5 Seated Mindful Breathing: Centering the Spirit

Sit comfortably, hands resting on your lap, and bring your attention to your breath. Inhale slowly, counting to four, and exhale, matching the count. Allow your breath to flow naturally, focusing on each inhalation and exhalation. If your mind wanders, gently guide it back to your breath. This Seated Mindful Breathing meditation serves as a centering practice, promoting a calm and present state of mind. Dedicate 5-10 minutes to this meditative journey.

5.2.6 Progressive Muscle Relaxation: Easing Tension

Remain seated and take a few deep breaths. Start with your toes, tensing and then releasing the muscles. Move progressively through each muscle group—calves, thighs, abdomen, shoulders, and so on—until you reach the muscles in your face. With each release, feel the tension melting away. Progressive Muscle Relaxation is a gentle technique to release physical and mental tension. Dedicate 10-15 minutes to this practice, savoring the deep relaxation that unfolds.

5.2.7 Chair Savasana: Restful Rejuvenation

Transition to a comfortable reclined position in your chair, arms resting by your sides. Close your eyes and allow your body to settle into the support of the chair. Focus on your breath, inhaling tranquility and exhaling any remaining tension. Chair Savasana offers a restful rejuvenation, creating space for a profound sense of peace. Savor this relaxation for 10-15 minutes, embracing the serenity that unfolds.

Cool Down and Guided Relaxation mark the culmination of your Chair Yoga practice, inviting you to surrender to the gentle embrace of tranquility. These meditation techniques for seniors are like whispers of peace, guiding you into a state of restful rejuvenation and providing a serene conclusion to your journey. As you bask in the stillness and serenity, may you find solace in the soothing rhythms of your breath and the quietude within.

Chapter 6: Two-Week Chair Yoga Plan

Week 1: Daily 10-Minute Chair Yoga Routines

Day 1: Seated Breath Awareness

- Begin in a comfortable seated position.
- Close your eyes and focus on your breath.
- Inhale deeply, feeling the expansion of your chest.
- Exhale slowly, releasing tension.
- Continue for 3-5 minutes, allowing the calming rhythm to center your mind.

Day 2: Neck and Shoulder Exercises

- Sit tall, shoulders relaxed.
- Inhale and exhale, gently tilting your head to the right.
- Inhale back to center and exhale, tilting to the left.
- Repeat for neck flexibility.
- Shrug your shoulders up and down for shoulder release.
- Perform each exercise for 10-15 seconds.

Day 3: Wrist and Ankle Circles

- Sit comfortably with feet flat.
- Circle your wrists clockwise, then counterclockwise.
- Lift your right foot, circle the ankle clockwise, then counterclockwise.
- Switch to the left foot.
- Repeat for joint flexibility.
- Perform each circle for 10-15 seconds.

Day 4: Seated Sun Salutations

- Inhale and reach your arms overhead.
- Exhale, bringing your hands to the heart center.
- Inhale to lift your arms again.
- Exhale to release them back down.
- Repeat for 2-3 minutes, flowing with breath.

Day 5: Seated Forward Bend Variations

- Begin in a seated position.
- Inhale and fold forward, reaching toward your feet.
- Hold for 30 seconds.
- Explore supported, one-legged, twisted, and shoulder-opener variations.
- Flow through the variations for 5 minutes.

Day 6: Seated Twist Sequence

- Sit with a tall spine.

- Inhale, twist to the right, placing the left hand on the right knee.
- Exhale back to center and repeat on the left side.
- Add shoulder opener and seated twist flow.
- Flow through the sequence for 5-7 minutes.

Day 7: Seated Warrior Poses

- Sit at the edge of the chair.
- Inhale, lifting your arms for Seated Warrior I.
- Exhale into Seated Warrior II.
- Inhale to Seated Warrior III, and exhale to Seated Reverse Warrior.
- Flow through the sequence, holding each pose for 30 seconds.
- Repeat on the other side.

Week 2: Daily 10-Minute Chair Yoga Routines

Day 8: Leg Lifts and Extensions Flow

- Sit tall with hands on the chair for support.
- Inhale for leg lift, exhale for extension.
- Switch legs in a flowing motion.
- Repeat for 5-7 minutes, engaging core and legs.

Day 9: Dynamic Chair Yoga Flow

- Start with Seated Cat-Cow Flow.
- Transition into Seated Sun Salutations.
- Flow into Seated Warrior Flow.
- Include Seated Twist and Reach.
- Conclude with Seated Forward Bend Flow.
- Repeat the sequence for 10 minutes.

Day 10: Chair-Assisted Standing Poses

- Begin with Chair Mountain Pose.
- Flow into Chair Tree Pose.
- Explore Chair Warrior Pose.
- Try Chair Dancer Pose with chair support.
- Conclude with Chair-Assisted Standing Forward Fold.
- Hold each pose for 30 seconds to 1 minute.

Day 11: Loving-Kindness Meditation

- Sit comfortably with your eyes closed.
- Inhale love for yourself, exhale love outward.
- Extend wishes of happiness, health, and ease.
- Expand wishes to others and all beings.
- Practice for 5-7 minutes.

Day 12: Seated Mindful Breathing

- Sit comfortably, hands on your lap.

- Inhale for a count of four, and exhale for a count of four.
- Focus on each breath, redirecting thoughts gently.
- Continue for 10 minutes, cultivating mindfulness.

Day 13: Progressive Muscle Relaxation

- Sit comfortably and close your eyes.
- Inhale and tense your toes, then exhale to release.
- Progressively move through muscle groups.
- Spend 15 minutes, allowing deep relaxation.

Day 14: Chair Savasana and Reflection

- Find a comfortable reclined position in your chair.
- Close your eyes, focus on your breath.
- Allow your body and mind to rest in Chair Savasana.
- Reflect on the two-week journey.
- Embrace the tranquility for 10-15 minutes.

Congratulations on completing the Two-Week Chair Yoga Plan! May the benefits of your practice continue to resonate in your daily life.

Chapter 7: Tips and FAQs

7.1 Modifying Poses for Individual Needs

Chair Yoga is a versatile practice that can be adapted to meet individual needs and abilities. Here are some tips for modifying poses:

Use Props: Introduce props like cushions or blocks to provide additional support and enhance comfort during poses.

Chair Height: Adjust the height of the chair to accommodate different body types and mobility levels. A higher chair may be preferable for those with knee or hip concerns.

Partial Movements: If a full range of motion is challenging, focus on partial movements within a pose. Gradually work towards the complete expression of the pose over time.

Seated Options: For standing poses, consider incorporating seated variations. This allows individuals with balance issues or discomfort to still experience the benefits of the pose.

Breathing Emphasis: Emphasize breath awareness and mindful breathing throughout the practice. Breathing is a fundamental aspect of yoga and can be practiced in any position.

Individual Consultation: For those with specific health concerns or limitations, consulting with a healthcare professional or a certified yoga instructor can provide personalized guidance for modifications.

Remember, the essence of Chair Yoga lies in making the practice accessible and enjoyable for everyone. Feel free to experiment with different modifications and find what works best for your unique needs.

7.2 Frequently Asked Questions (FAQs)

Q1: Can Chair Yoga be practiced by individuals with limited mobility?

A1: Absolutely! Chair Yoga is designed to cater to individuals with a wide range of mobility levels. The practice can be adapted to accommodate those with limited mobility, making it a suitable option for individuals seeking a gentle and accessible form of exercise.

Q2: Is Chair Yoga only for seniors?

A2: While Chair Yoga is often associated with seniors, it is inclusive and suitable for individuals of all ages. The practice can be beneficial for anyone looking to improve flexibility, strength, and overall well-being, regardless of age.

Q3: How often should Chair Yoga be practiced?

A3: The frequency of Chair Yoga practice can vary based on individual preferences and schedules. Starting with a few sessions per week and gradually increasing as comfort and interest grow is a good approach. Consistency is key, even if it's just a few minutes each day.

Q4: Can Chair Yoga help with stress reduction?

A4: Yes, Chair Yoga can be an effective tool for stress reduction. The combination of gentle movements, focused breathing, and mindfulness creates a calming effect on the nervous system, promoting relaxation and stress relief.

Q5: Are there any specific clothing or equipment requirements for Chair Yoga?

A5: Comfortable and loose-fitting clothing is recommended for ease of movement. The only piece of equipment needed is a sturdy chair without arms. Props such as cushions or blocks can be added for support and comfort.

Q6: Can Chair Yoga be done at the office or during work breaks?

A6: Absolutely! Chair Yoga offers a convenient option for incorporating movement and relaxation into a busy workday. Simple stretches and breathing exercises can be done at a desk or in a break area to alleviate tension and improve focus.

Q7: How can Chair Yoga benefit individuals with chronic conditions?

A7: Chair Yoga can be adapted to accommodate various chronic conditions, providing a gentle form of exercise. The practice may help improve flexibility, reduce pain, and enhance overall well-being. However, individuals with chronic conditions should consult with their healthcare provider before starting any new exercise routine.

Remember, these FAQs provide general information, and individual experiences may vary. It's always advisable to consult with a healthcare professional before beginning a new exercise program, especially for those with pre-existing health conditions. Enjoy the journey of Chair Yoga and explore how it can be uniquely tailored to meet your needs.

Conclusion

As we draw the final curtain on this odyssey of Chair Yoga, I invite you to reflect on the whispers of transformation that have unfolded within the intimate embrace of your chair. In the tapestry of these pages, you've navigated the ebb and flow of breath, surrendered to the dance of movement, and found solace in the stillness. It's not merely a practice; it's a journey—a journey that transcends the confines of physical postures and transcends into the realm of empowerment, self-discovery, and well-being.

Your chair, once a mundane companion in the ordinary rhythm of life, has now become a vessel of empowerment. It witnessed your commitment, felt the cadence of your breath, and cradled you in moments of introspection. Through each pose, each breath, and each stretch, you unfolded a new chapter within the book of your own body and soul.

In the world of Chair Yoga, your limitations are transformed into gateways of possibility. The chair, a humble prop, became the conduit through which you rediscovered the language of your body—a language that speaks of strength, flexibility, and resilience. The chair witnessed your metamorphosis, from the initial trepidation to the graceful flow of a well-practiced sequence.

Yet, beyond the physicality, Chair Yoga beckons you to a sacred space—a space where mindfulness intertwined with movement, where breath became a bridge between the tangible and the ethereal. In this space, you unearthed the power of presence, the art of letting go, and the beauty of embracing each moment with a mindful heart.

As you close this chapter, know that your journey doesn't end here. It merely transforms, becoming a companion on the ongoing expedition of your well-being. The chair, once a prop, now stands as a symbol—a symbol of empowerment, of resilience, of the infinite potential residing within.

May the wisdom woven into these pages accompany you as you carry the essence of Chair Yoga into your daily life. May each stretch remind you of your inherent strength, each breath anchor you to the present, and each moment of stillness be a reminder of the boundless peace that resides within.

Thank you for entrusting your practice to these words. May your journey beyond these pages be a continued exploration of self-discovery, empowerment, and the limitless possibilities that await within the sacred embrace of your chair.

Namaste.

Appendix: Illustrated Pose Guide

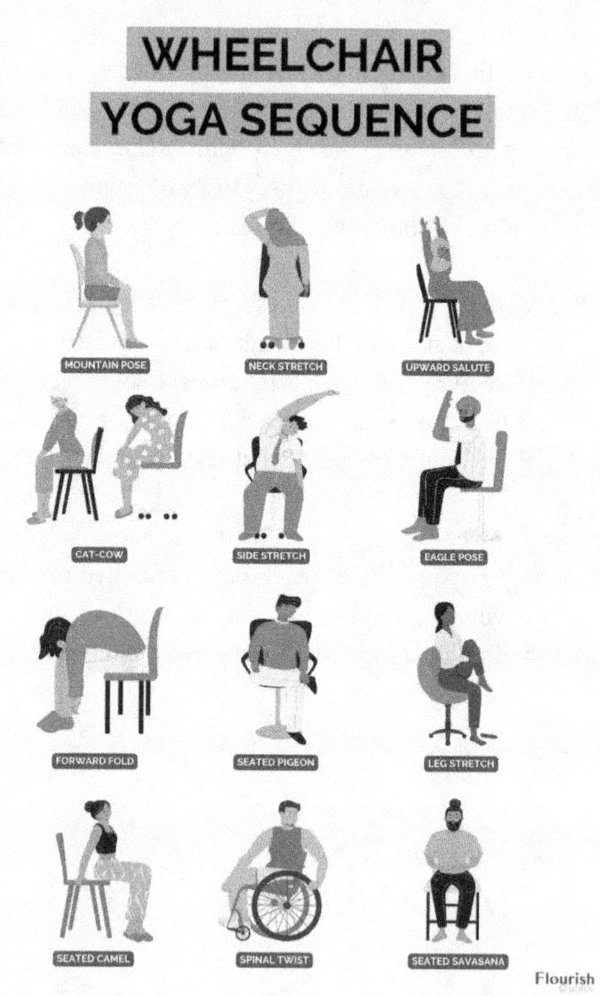

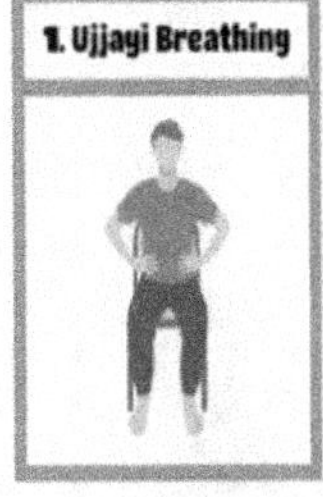
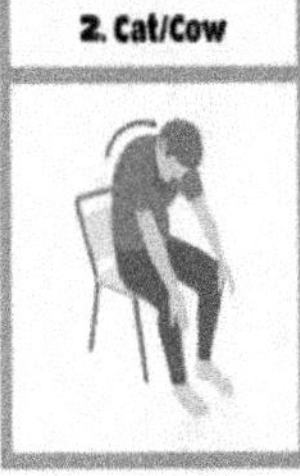
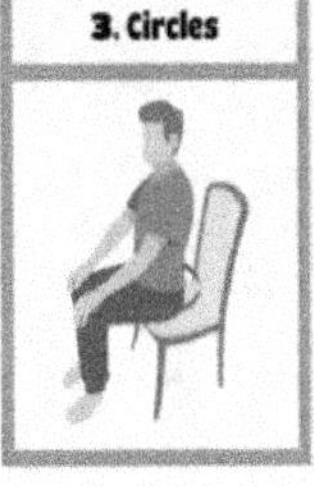
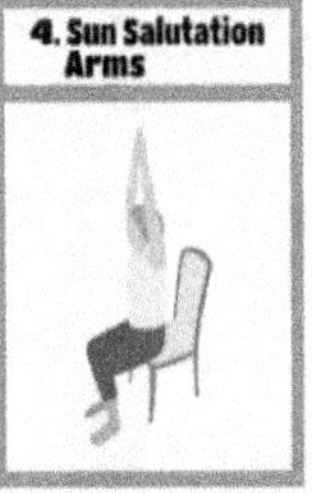
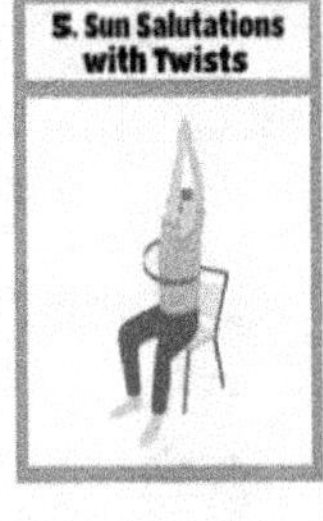
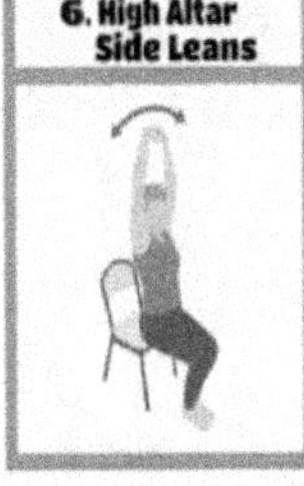
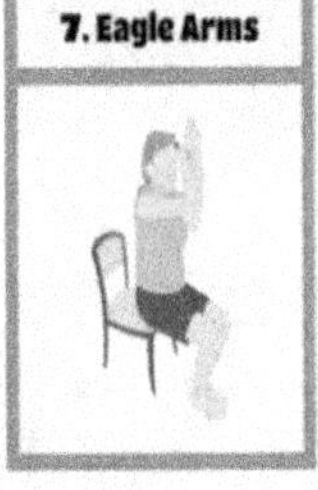
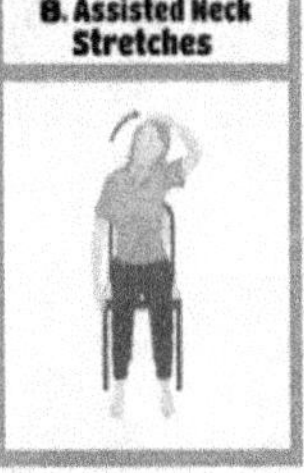
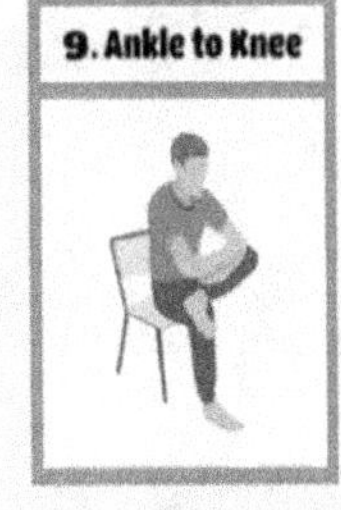
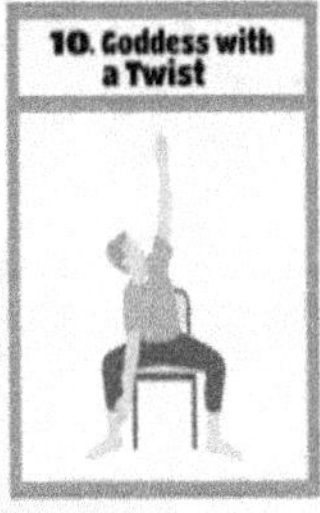
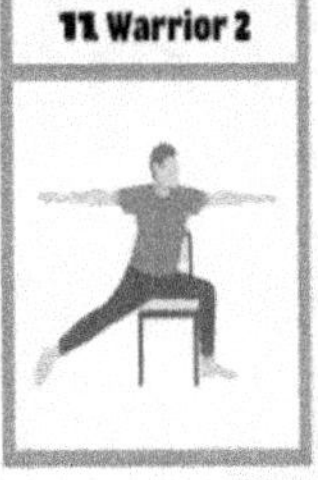
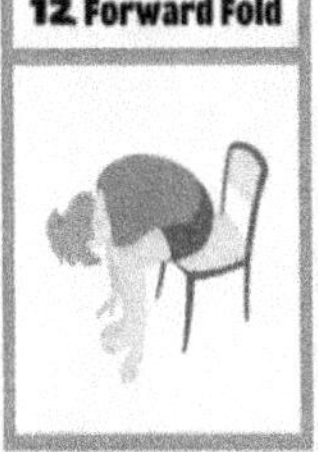

SENIOR CHAIR YOGA POSES
1. Ujjayi Breathing
2. Cat/Cow
3. Circles
4. Sun Salutation Arms
5. Sun Salutations with Twists
6. High Altar Side Leans
7. Eagle Arms
8. Assisted Neck Stretches
9. Ankle to Knee
10. Goddess with a Twist
11. Warrior 2
12. Forward Fold

— SEATED SUN SALUTATIONS —

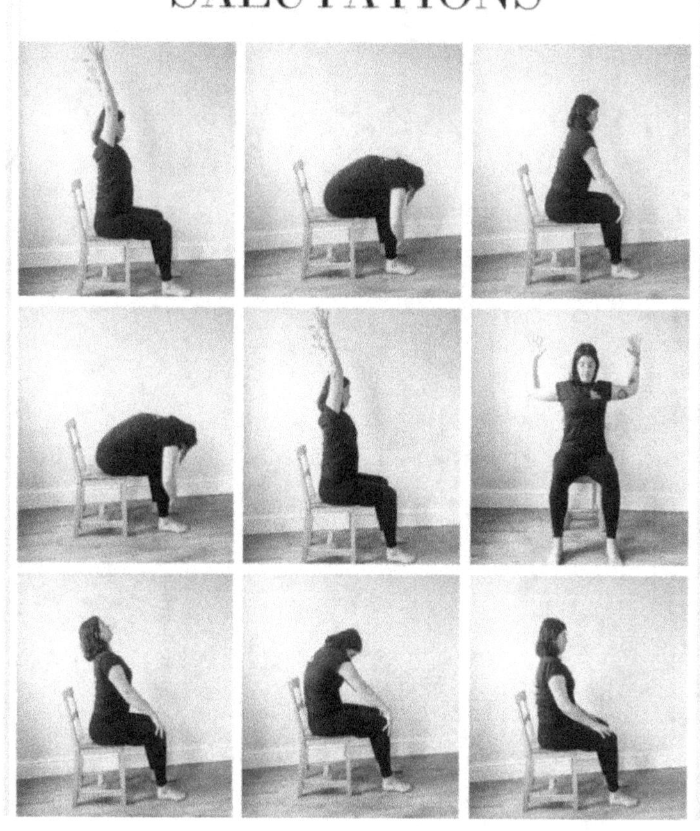

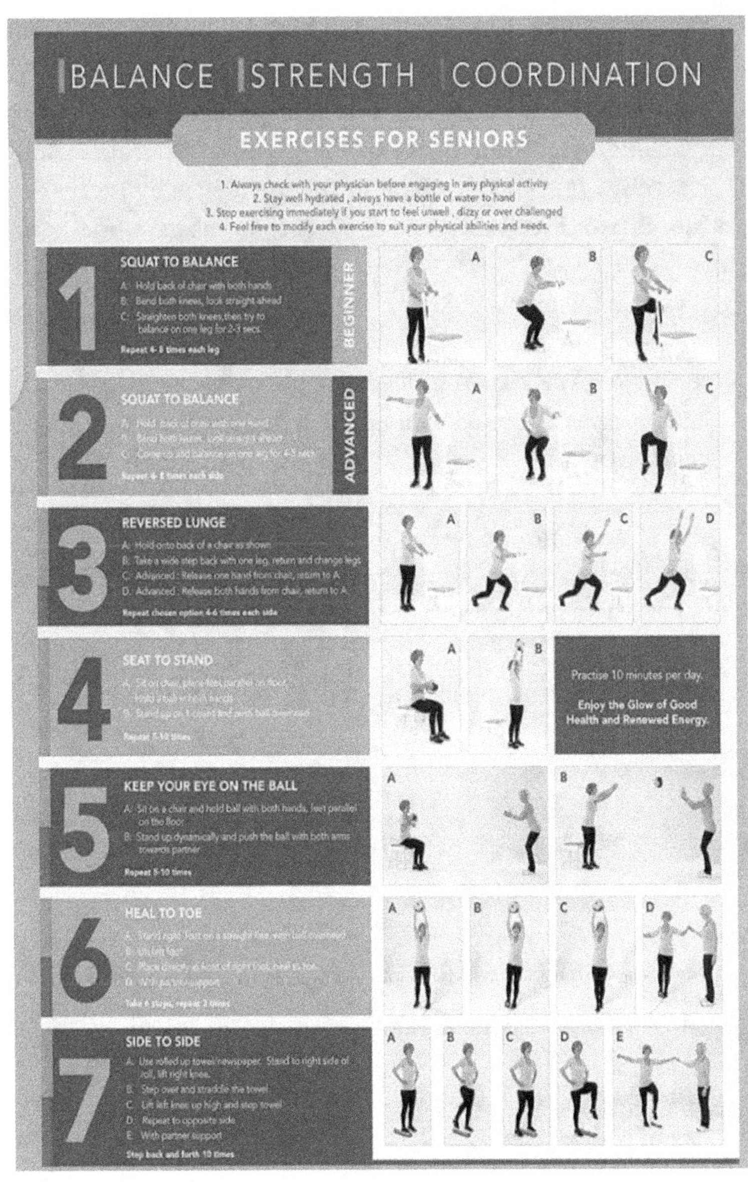

BALANCE STRENGTH COORDINATION
EXERCISES FOR SENIORS
1. Always check with your physician before engaging in any physical activity
2. Stay well hydrated , always have a bottle of water to hand
3. Stop exercising immediately if you start to feel unwell , dizzy or over challenged
4. Feel free to modify each exercise to suit your physical abilities and needs.
1
SQUAT TO BALANCE
A: Hold back of chair with both hands
B: Bend both knees, look straight ahead
C: Straighten both knees, then try to balance on one leg for 2-3 secs
Repeat 4- 6 times each leg
BEGINNER
A B C
2
SQUAT TO BALANCE
A: Hold back of chair with one hand
B: Bend both knees, look straight ahead
C: Come up and balance on one leg for 4-5 secs
Repeat 4- 6 times each side
ADVANCED
A B C
3
REVERSED LUNGE
A: Hold onto back of a chair as shown
B: Take a wide step back with one leg, return and change legs
C: Advanced : Release one hand from chair, return to A
D: Advanced : Release both hands from chair, return to A
Repeat chosen option 4-6 times each side
A B C D
4
SEAT TO STAND
A: Sit on chair, place feet parallel on floor, hold a ball with both hands
B: Stand up on 1 count and push ball overhead
Repeat 5-10 times
A B
Practise 10 minutes per day.
Enjoy the Glow of Good Health and Renewed Energy.
5
KEEP YOUR EYE ON THE BALL
A: Sit on a chair and hold ball with both hands, feet parallel on the floor
B: Stand up dynamically and push the ball with both arms towards partner
Repeat 5-10 times
A B
6
HEAL TO TOE
A: Stand right foot on a straight line with left overhead
B: Lift left foot
C: Place directly in front of right foot, heel to toe
D: With partner support
Take 6 steps, repeat 3 times
A B C D
7
SIDE TO SIDE
A: Use rolled up towel/newspaper. Stand to right side of roll, lift right knee.
B: Step over and straddle the towel
C: Lift left knee up high and step towel
D: Repeat to opposite side
E: With partner support
Step back and forth 10 times
A B C D E

Dear Readers,

We want to express our heartfelt gratitude for choosing **"Chair Yoga For Seniors Over 60: Quick 10-Minute Chair Exercises for Seniors - Regain Independence by Increasing Mobility & Flexibility."** Your support means the world to us.

If you've found this guide beneficial on your wellness journey, we kindly request you to take a moment to leave a positive review on Amazon. Your feedback not only encourages us but also inspires others to explore the transformative potential of chair yoga.

Thank you for being a part of our community and for investing in your well-being. Your success stories and experiences are the driving force behind our mission.

With sincere appreciation,
  Krista Bonds.

www.ingramcontent.com/pod-product-compliance
Lightning Source LLC
Chambersburg PA
CBHW060806260726
48660CB00002B/800